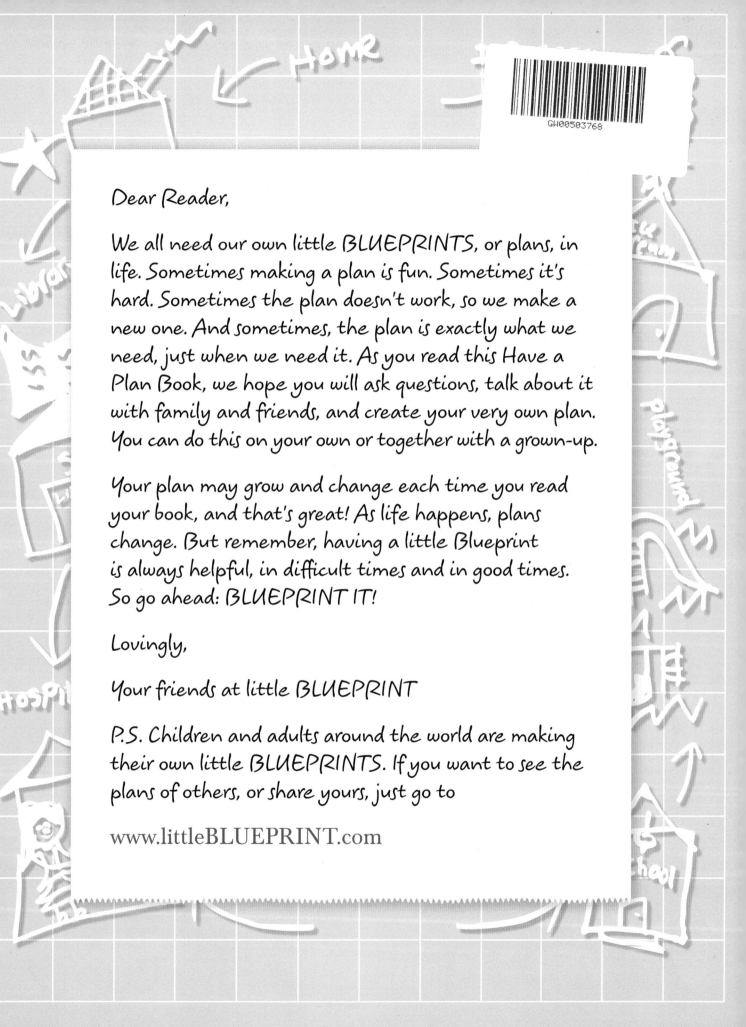

Dear Reader,

We all need our own little BLUEPRINTS, or plans, in life. Sometimes making a plan is fun. Sometimes it's hard. Sometimes the plan doesn't work, so we make a new one. And sometimes, the plan is exactly what we need, just when we need it. As you read this Have a Plan Book, we hope you will ask questions, talk about it with family and friends, and create your very own plan. You can do this on your own or together with a grown-up.

Your plan may grow and change each time you read your book, and that's great! As life happens, plans change. But remember, having a little Blueprint is always helpful, in difficult times and in good times. So go ahead: BLUEPRINT IT!

Lovingly,

Your friends at little BLUEPRINT

P.S. Children and adults around the world are making their own little BLUEPRINTS. If you want to see the plans of others, or share yours, just go to

www.littleBLUEPRINT.com

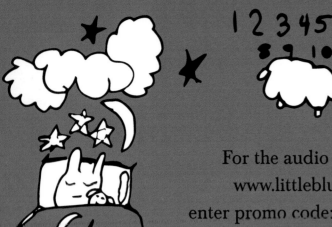
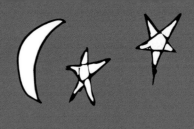
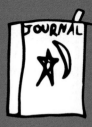

For the audio download, please go to:
www.littleblueprint.com/download
enter promo code: LB4000-654GF-BEDTIME

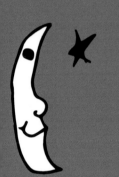

HAVE A PLAN *Books*

To purchase a hardcover or
personalized version of any
little BLUEPRINT book,
with names, optional photo(s),
and details, please go to:

www.littleBLUEPRINT.com

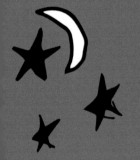

The author would like to thank,
for all of their support and expertise:
Dan Siegel, M.D.;
Nina Shapiro, M.D.; and
my editors, Leslie Budnick and Gina Shaw.
A special thanks to:
JAGA; and
Phoebe, age 10, for her blueprint and title page illustrations.

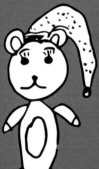
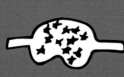
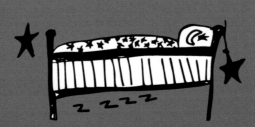
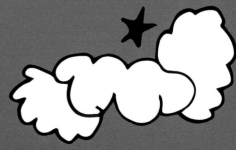

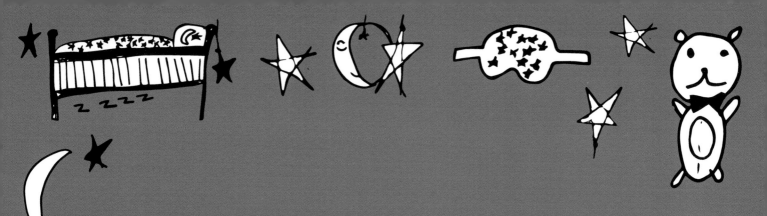

WHEN IT'S TIME
for Bed,
I HAVE A PLAN

by Katherine Eskovitz

illustrated by Jessica Churchill

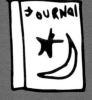
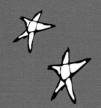

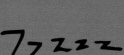
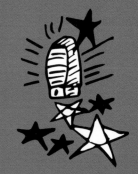
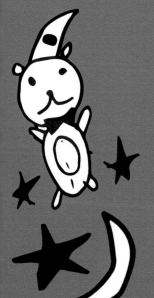
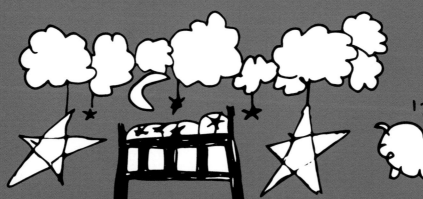

One thing I can tell you about myself:

Sometimes, I do **NOT** like to go to bed.

Or at least MY BRAIN TELLS MY BODY it does not

want to go to bed.

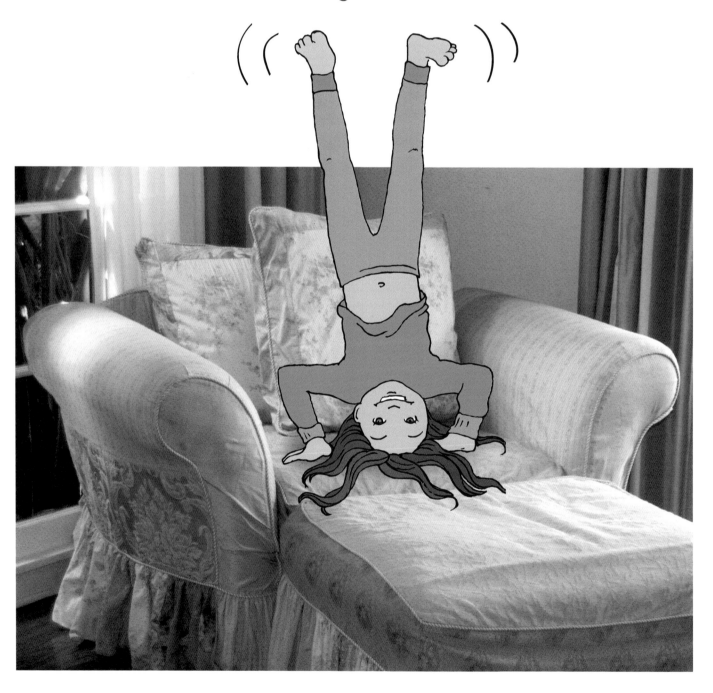

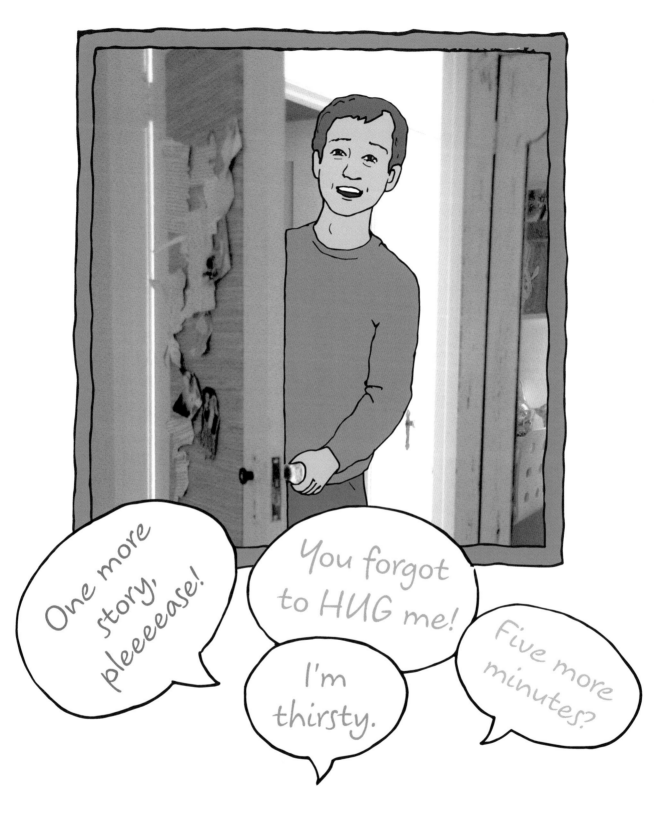

I just have one more question . . .

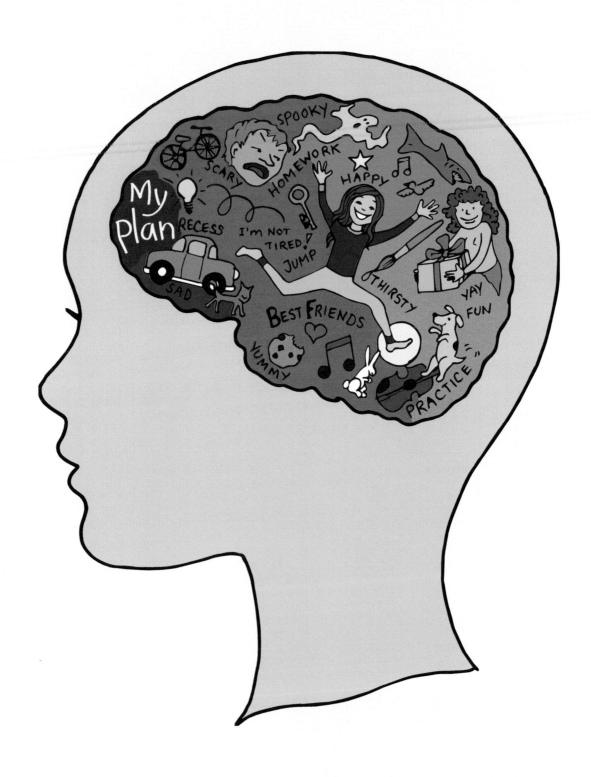

My brain might tell my body it is not tired,
but my body **NEEDS** rest even when it doesn't feel tired.

And since I am the boss of my brain,

I can talk to my brain and help it

RELAX MY BODY,

AND CALM MY MIND,

so I can have a cozy night's sleep.

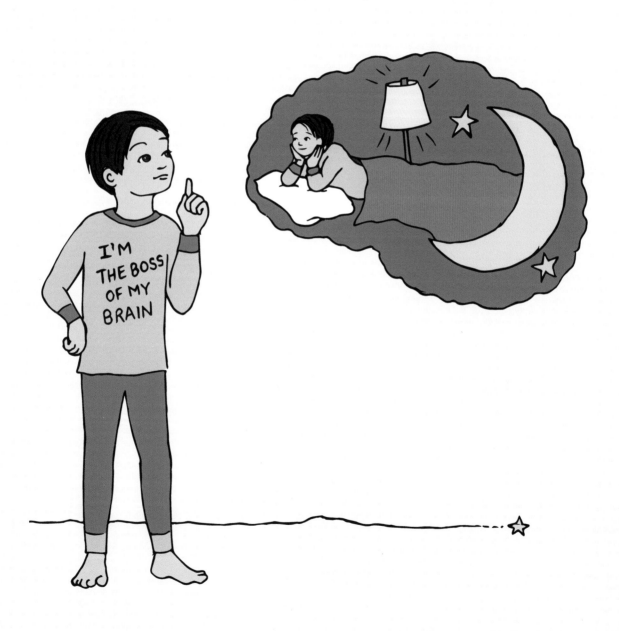

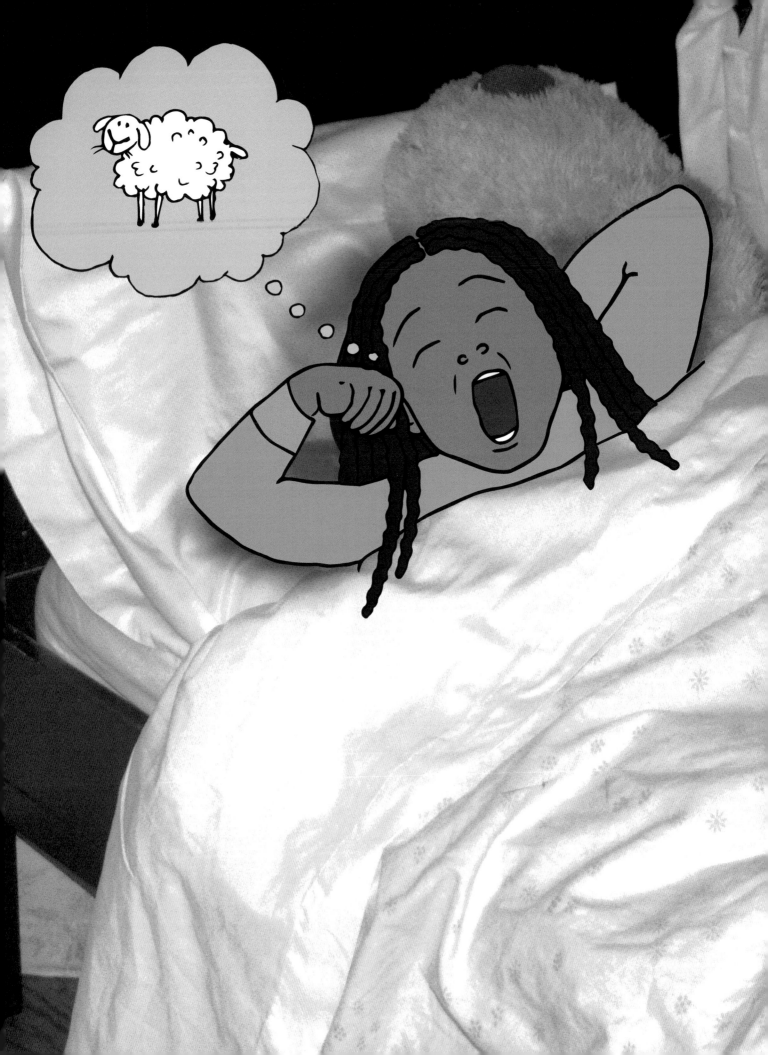

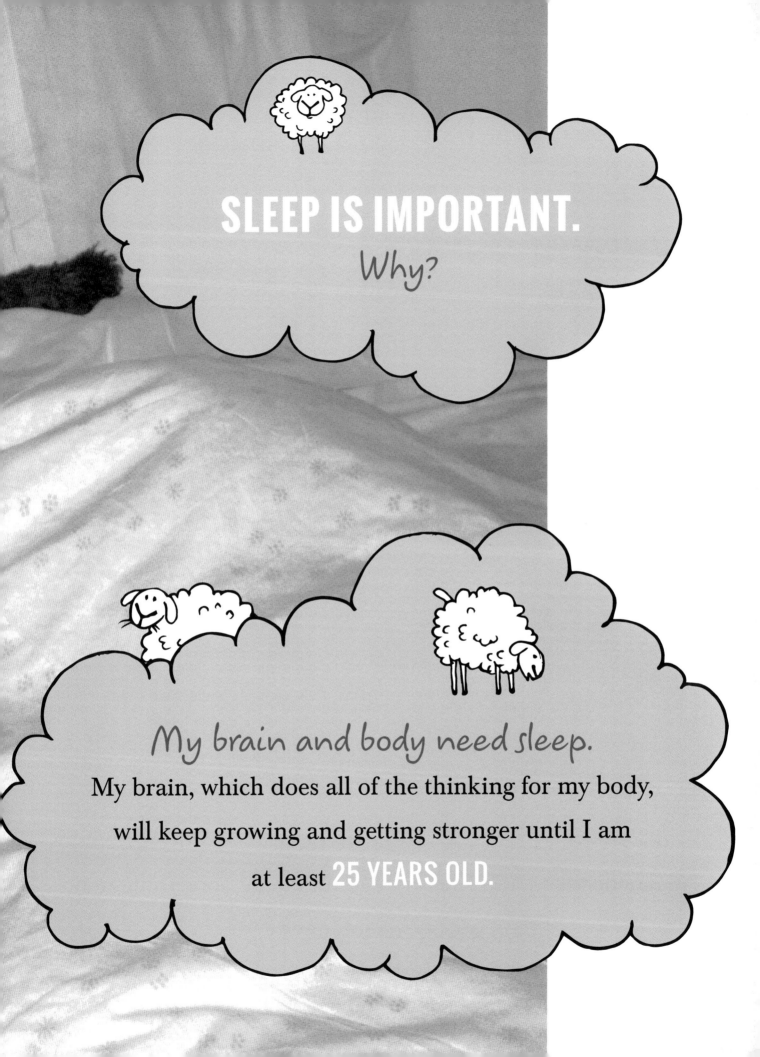

SLEEP IS IMPORTANT.

Why?

My brain and body need sleep.

My brain, which does all of the thinking for my body,
will keep growing and getting stronger until I am
at least **25 YEARS OLD.**

My brain is always working.

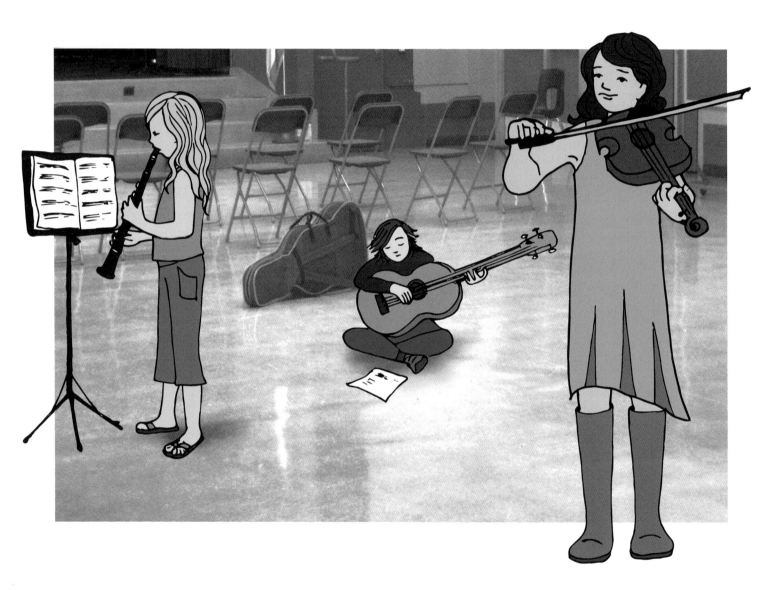

When I **PRACTICE** something over and over,
make mistakes, and then try again to learn something new,
I am strengthening my **BRAIN**.

It's the same with my BODY.
With practice, my body and brain
grow stronger and learn new things.

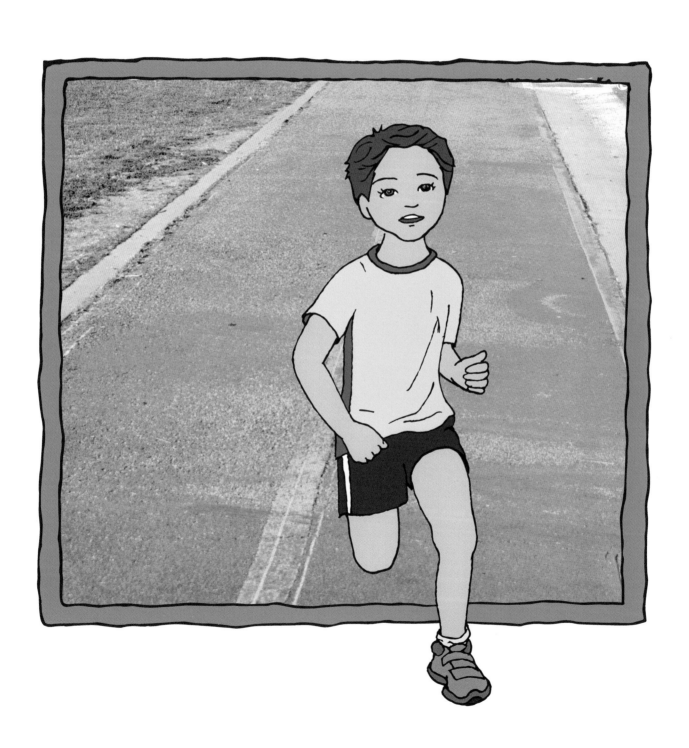

But another important way to strengthen my brain and body is by doing the OPPOSITE of practice and hard work: NOTHING. Well, almost nothing: SLEEPING.

Sleeping is one of the most important ways to strengthen my brain and body.

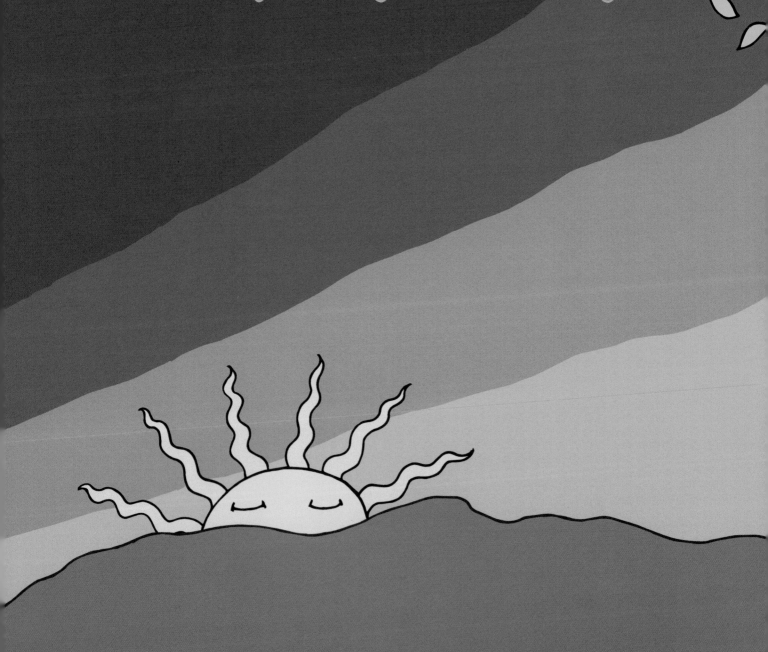

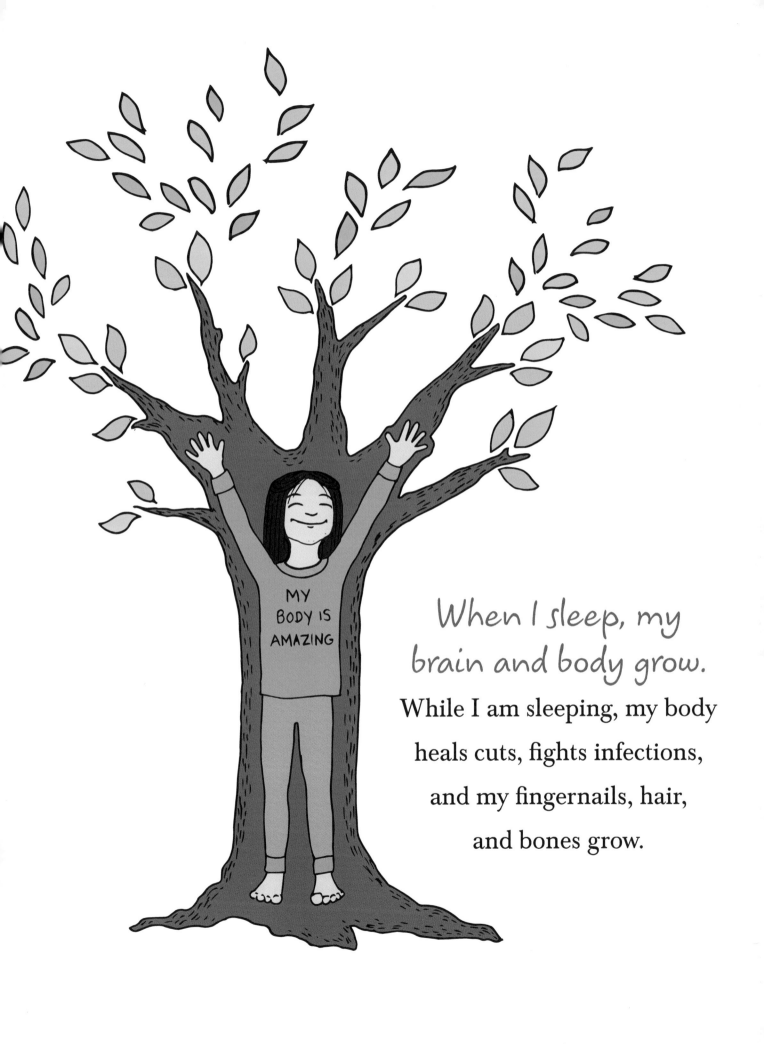

When I sleep, my brain and body grow. While I am sleeping, my body heals cuts, fights infections, and my fingernails, hair, and bones grow.

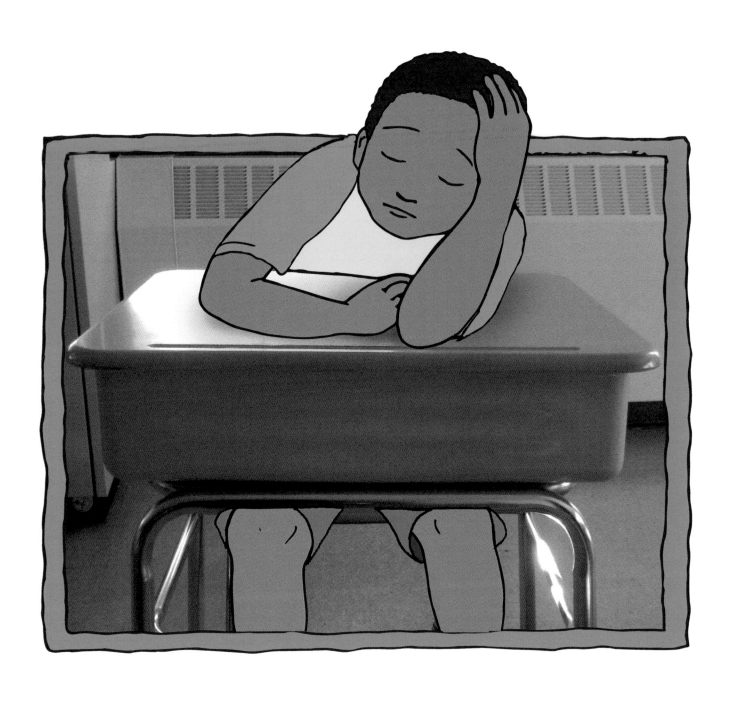

When I don't get enough sleep,

I can get sick more easily,

it can take longer to get better,

and my brain cannot think clearly.

Sometimes when I'm TIRED,
I feel teary or grouchy.

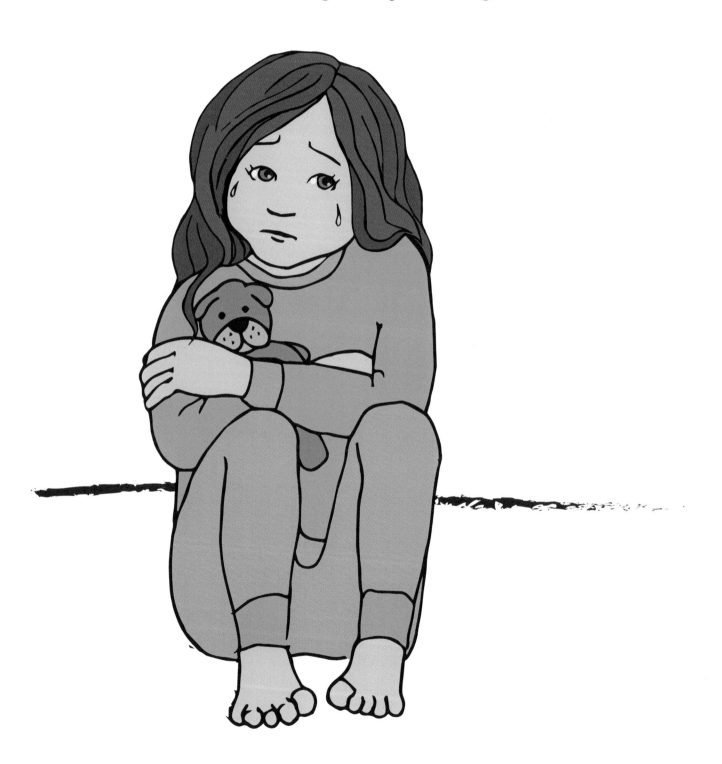

Do I get enough sleep?

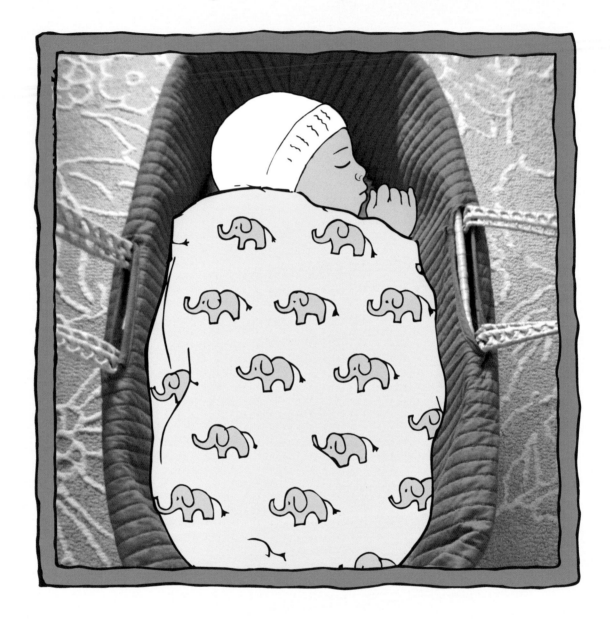

When I was a baby, I slept most of the time.
Before the age of 5, we need at least 12 hours
of sleep every night. From ages 5 to 12, we still need
10 TO 11 HOURS OF SLEEP EACH NIGHT.
Even teenagers need about 9 hours of sleep.

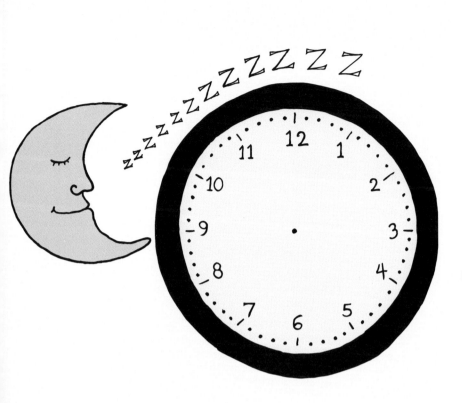

I can draw the time
I go to bed,
and the time I wake up.

I can count the hours

between when I GO TO BED and when I WAKE UP

to see if I am getting ENOUGH SLEEP.

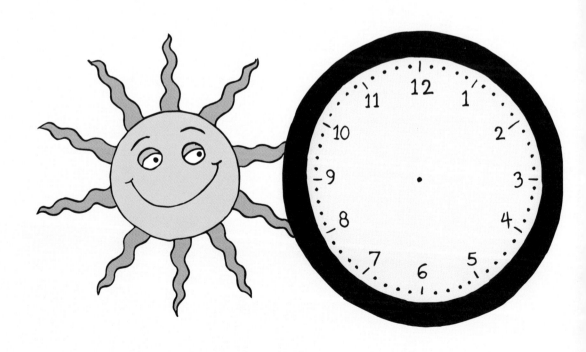

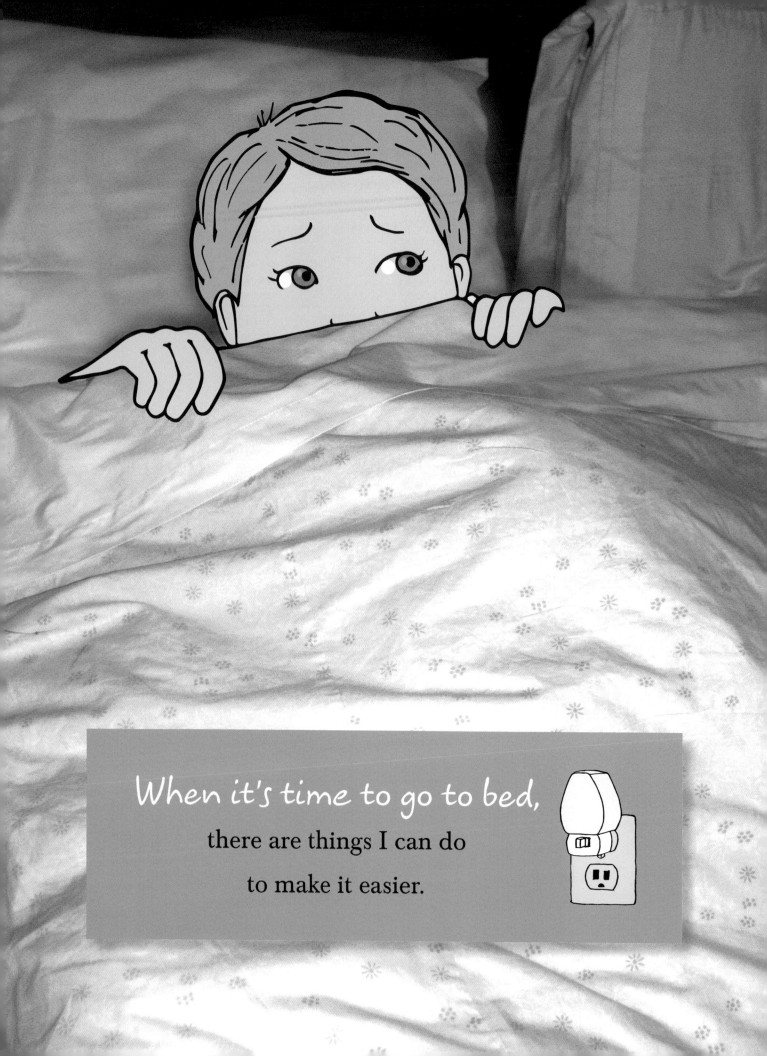

When it's time to go to bed, there are things I can do to make it easier.

I can create a bedtime plan.
CHOOSING QUIET ACTIVITIES,
RELAXING MY MIND,
AND DIMMING THE LIGHTS
before bedtime help teach my brain it is time for sleep.

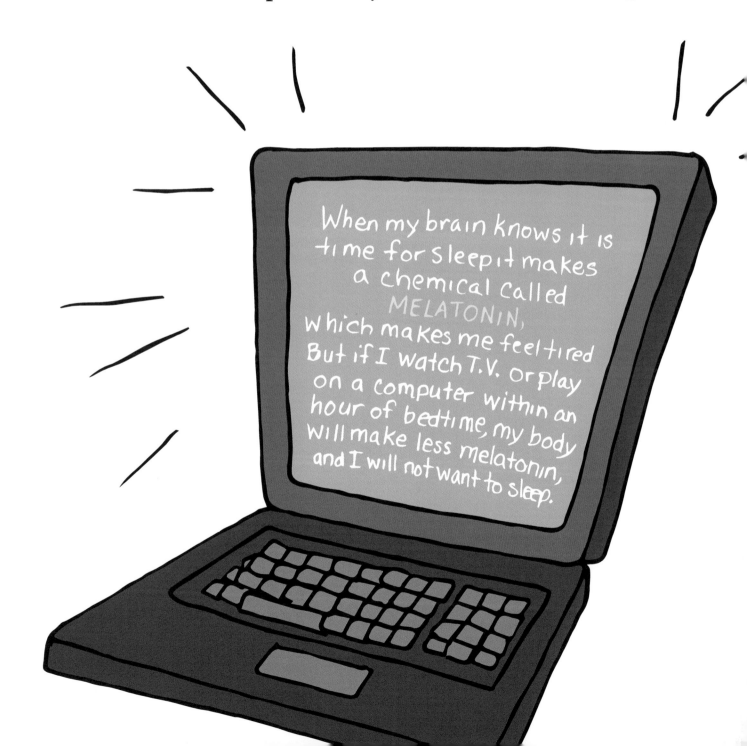

When my brain knows it is time for sleep it makes a chemical called MELATONIN, which makes me feel tired. But if I watch T.V. or play on a computer within an hour of bedtime, my body will make less melatonin, and I will not want to sleep.

I can start a Good-Night Journal.

For a few minutes each night before bedtime,
I can WRITE or DRAW anything I want.
This can clear and calm my brain.

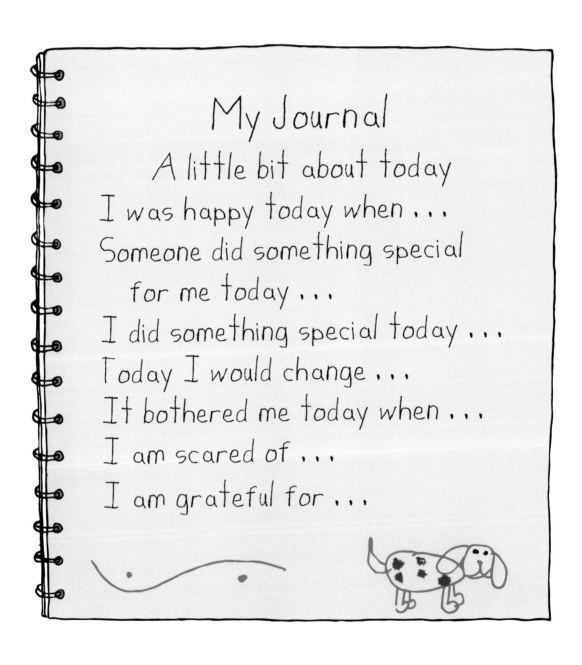

My Journal
A little bit about today
I was happy today when . . .
Someone did something special
    for me today . . .
I did something special today . . .
Today I would change . . .
It bothered me today when . . .
I am scared of . . .
I am grateful for . . .

I can play a short bedtime game
while we dim the lights and lie in bed.

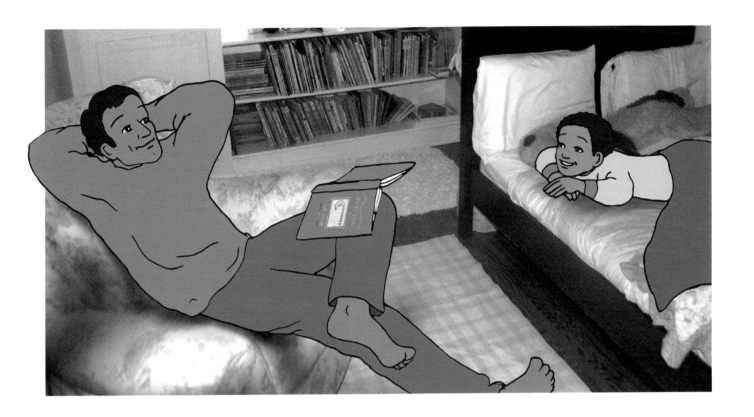

ONE FUN GAME IS TWO TRUTHS AND ONE FAKE:
We take turns telling two things we really did that day,
and one thing we did not do, then see if the other person
can guess which thing is made up.

This is an amusing way to TALK ABOUT OUR DAY
and help RELAX OUR BRAINS.

Good Night, Dear Brain (yawn), Good Night . . .

I can close my eyes and listen to
"Good Night, Dear Brain (yawn), Good Night."
I can even record my own good-night talk or
play soothing music to listen to before bedtime.

Because I am the boss of my brain

I can imagine whatever I want to fall asleep.

I can picture myself comfy in my safe, cozy bed.

If I am scared to go to bed one night, or I have a bad dream,

I can change SCARY THOUGHTS into SILLY THOUGHTS.

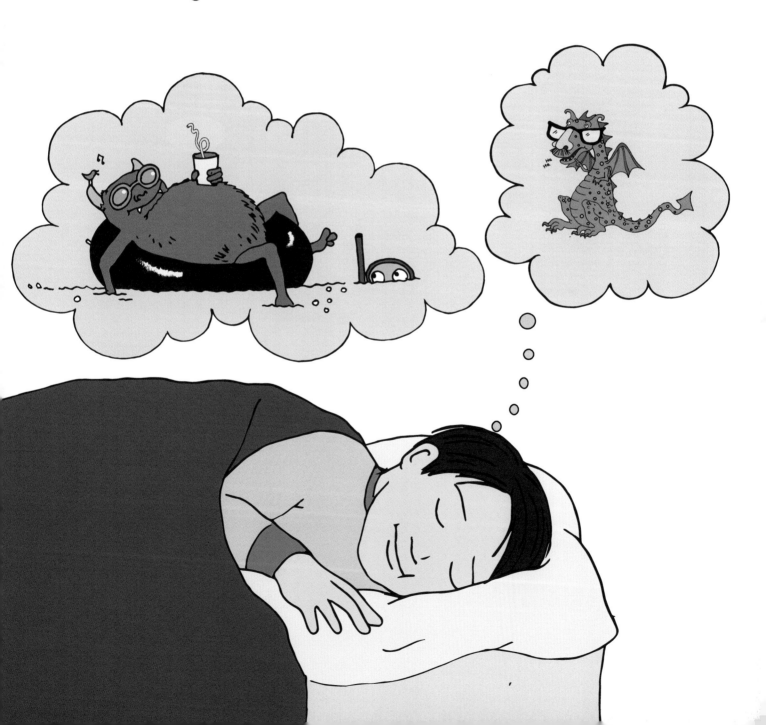

I can remind my brain that
someone special is always there for me,
even while I am sleeping.

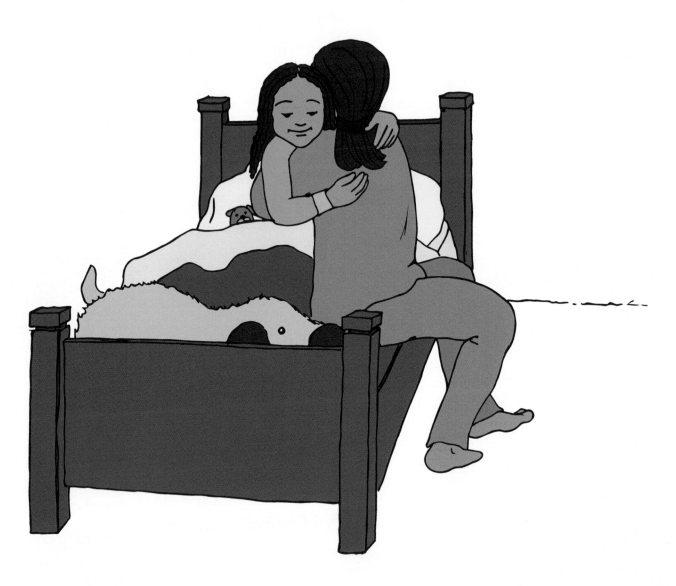

After I give a good-night hug, I can cuddle with my
FAVORITE STUFFED ANIMAL as I fall asleep.

I can teach my brain to have a cozy night's sleep by using the ideas in this book to make my very own plan.

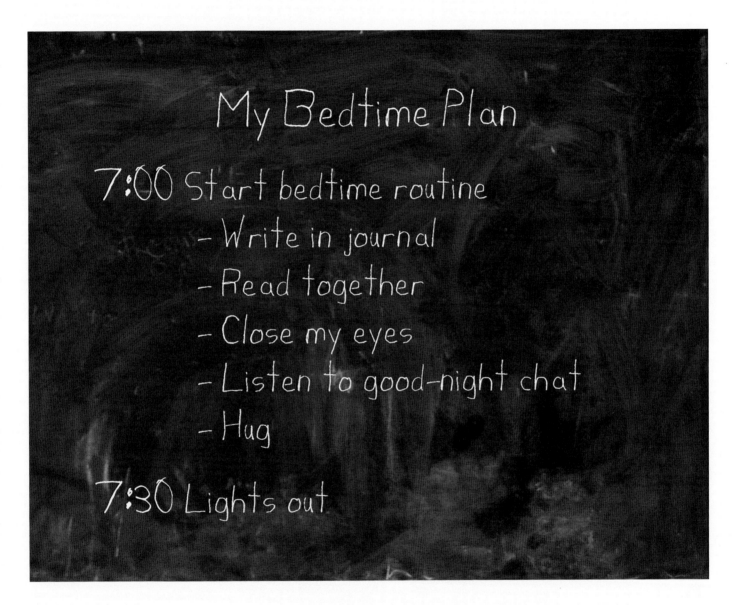

My Bedtime Plan

7:00 Start bedtime routine
— Write in journal
— Read together
— Close my eyes
— Listen to good-night chat
— Hug

7:30 Lights out

Whatever I choose, it is important that I try to follow the SAME PLAN and go to bed at the SAME TIME each night, so my brain knows it is time to be sleepy.

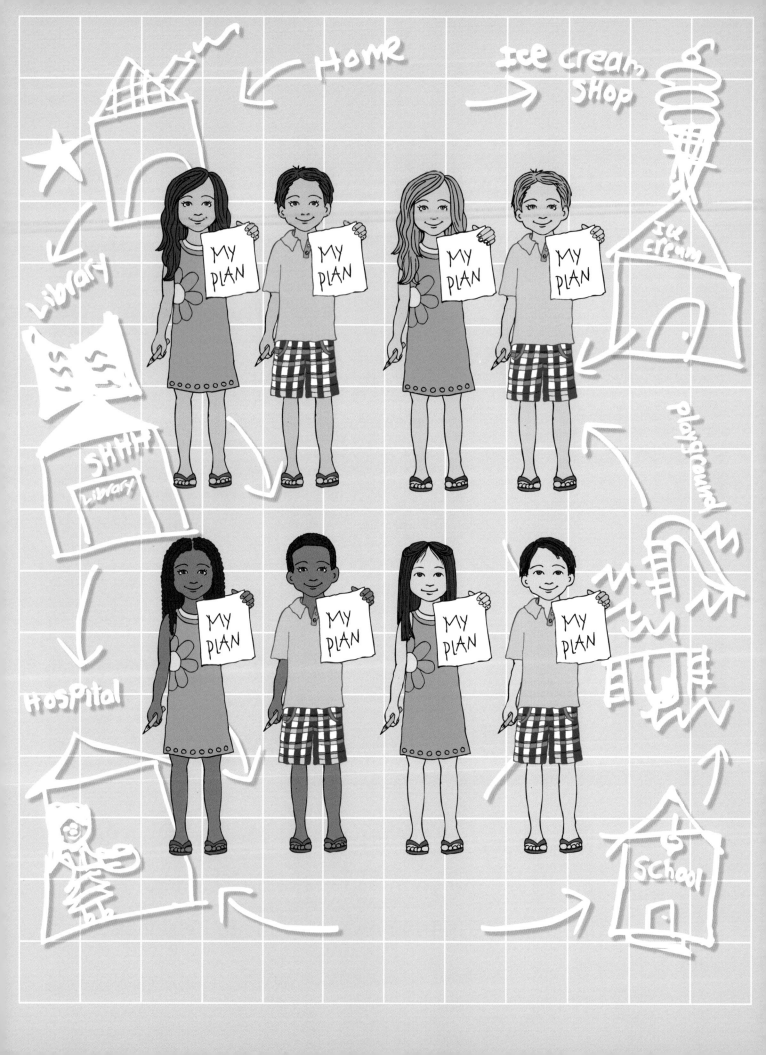

Here is MY PLAN

Check out other children's BLUEPRINTS from around the world and share yours, too!

Other titles in the
HAVE A PLAN Series

TO BE A HEALTHY EATER, I HAVE A PLAN

TO CELEBRATE THE HOLIDAYS, I HAVE A PLAN

WHEN I MISS SOMEONE SPECIAL, I HAVE A PLAN

WHEN I MISS MY SPECIAL PET, I HAVE A PLAN

TO BE SAFE AT HOME, I HAVE A PLAN

TO BE SAFE ON THE GO, I HAVE A PLAN

TO KEEP MY BODY SAFE, I HAVE A PLAN

WHEN MY PARENTS DIVORCE, I HAVE A PLAN

WHEN MY PARENTS SEPARATE, I HAVE A PLAN

AND MORE

New titles added regularly at

www.littleBLUEPRINT.com

All titles are available ready-made and personalized

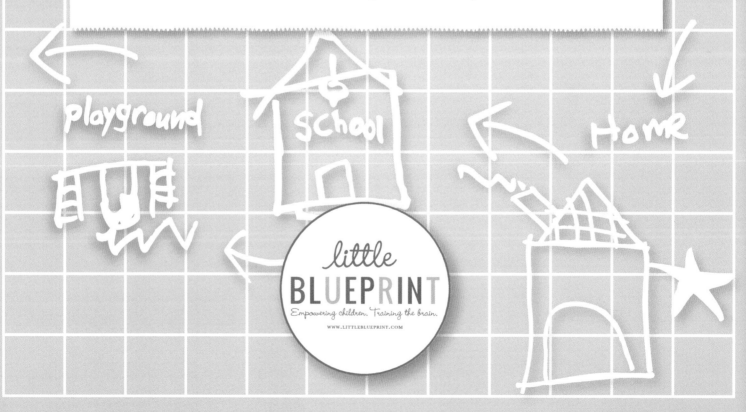

Printed in Great Britain
by Amazon